The Little Diabetes
Book of Common Sense

The Little Diabetes Book of Common Sense

A Can-Do Program for Managing or Preventing Type 2 Diabetes

Carol J. Flick Wright, RN,CDE
Certified Diabetes Educator

The Little Diabetes Book of Common Sense
Title ID: 6364204
Copyright © 2016 Carol J. Flick Wright, RN,CDE
All rights reserved.
ISBN: 1534828974
ISBN 13: 9781534828971

Contents

Endorsements

This short, direct, clearly stated and easily understood book is certain to be a useful and possibly lifesaving tool for those with type 2 diabetes or prediabetes.

Ms. Wright has presented the problem and the solution in terms anyone can easily understand. This should be required reading for anyone at risk for diabetes.

—Howard M. Haft, MD, MMM, CPE, FACPE
Deputy Secretary of Public Health at the Maryland Department of Health and Mental Hygiene

I think the book is great. Carol presents a very complicated topic in a way that patients can easily understand. Good Work.

—Meindert Smith, MD
Specialist Internal Medicine

I have read your transcript, and I think you have done a wonderful job. What a wake-up call I had when I was diagnosed with diabetes. The common-sense approach, as you describe it in your book, reminds me of the "for dummies" books that have always attracted this dummy at the local bookstore. I have always liked the phrase that "you don't know what you don't know." I knew nothing about diabetes until I was diagnosed with this disease.

You have laid it all out for those who care to care about their physical well-being. You have "set the table" for those who wish to follow a simple carbohydrate diet and exercise program to treat diabetes. It is also important to have an accountability partner. Paula, my wife, has almost finished reading your book, and she has become my accountability partner.

Your book should do very well. I want to thank you for giving me the opportunity to have one of the first reads.

—Bob Harry, Patient

What an amazing book! It is exactly what we need, because everything is explained so clearly, and you answered all the key questions that I as an accountability partner needed to know.
It is a perfect reference book for the whole family! Thank you so much for sharing this with us.

—Paula Harry, Spouse

I read the book and found it very informative. I liked it very much. I think people who read it will really understand what having diabetes does to their body and how to eat. Great book!

—Eileen Di Poli, RN and Patient

This book is dedicated to Ann Crispin, an author and patient who became a dearly loved friend. Thank you, Ann, for inspiring me to write this book and for haunting me until I completed it. You are an *awesome* muse!

Preface

In the early 1990s, I worked as a home health nurse in rural southern Maryland. More than fifty percent of my patients were suffering from the devastating effects of complications from type 2 diabetes. At that time, medical professionals anticipated complications as part of the disease's natural course.

When the results of the Diabetes Control and Complications Trial (DCCT) came out in 1993, the medical community began to understand that diabetes complications could be prevented by keeping blood sugar in good control (an A1C of <7%). Because diabetes is a self-management disease, it became evident that diabetes self-management education was the most important element of living well with type 2 diabetes. In those days, a patient typically saw his or her doctor four to twelve times a year; the rest of the time, the patient was responsible for his own health. Patients *needed* to know about diabetes.

Urine testing for sugar gave way to cumbersome, yet more accurate, blood-glucose meters. Meters became more user friendly, and patients were eager to learn how to live well with diabetes. More and more diabetes medications became available. Self-management programs began to spring up all over the nation.

People who had diabetes began to realize that if they wanted to prevent complications and live the healthiest life possible, they were going to have to find out how to self-manage their diagnosis.

In 1994, I developed and implemented a self-management health-education program for a large internal-medicine and family-practice group. I became a certified diabetes educator in 1996 and I have been helping people live well with diabetes ever since.

In 2002, the results of the Diabetes Prevention Program (DPP) were released, and we realized type 2 diabetes can be prevented or delayed if patients are identified *before* the blood sugar reaches a diagnostic level for type 2 diabetes. Patients must choose to make some simple lifestyle changes to prevent the development of full-blown diabetes. This requires their being able to learn how to keep themselves healthy and diabetes-free.

In the past two decades, I have helped more than two thousand people avoid the complications of type 2 diabetes by ensuring they understand their disease and understand what their choices are to help them avoid the devastating complications of type 2 diabetes.

This book will not make it possible for the reader to pass a pathology or physiology course in diabetes; diabetes is an intricate and complicated disease that is still being studied.

This book *will*, however, make it possible for the reader to personally understand the disease, understand the choices available to him or her, and understand how best to prevent complications.

I have written this book as though the reader were sitting on my office sofa and we were sharing ways in which he or she could best live well with diabetes. I use what I call "mind pictures" to help my patients grasp the depth of the ruthlessness and devastation that accompany *unmanaged* diabetes.

I hope you enjoy reading *The Little Diabetes Book of Common Sense* as much as I have enjoyed sharing these principles with my patients during the past twenty years.

It works if you work it!

A Wake-Up Call

I recently saw my cousin, Sue, whom I had not seen for more than five years. She was *radiant*; she looked beautiful and vibrant. I said, "Sue, you become more beautiful with each birthday. How do you do it?"

"I got my wake-up call a couple of years ago when I was diagnosed with type 2 diabetes," Sue explained. She had learned healthy eating, healthy exercising, and healthy ways to manage stress. As a result, she'd lost fifty pounds, and life was rosy.

Sue is a school teacher who, before her diagnosis, had been thinking of retiring; she was always tired, had very little motivation, and felt she was "just getting old." But with her newfound energy and vitality, she told me, "I still have kids who need me!"

Now Sue has *no* plans for impending retirement, and she says she feels better than she has in twenty years!

Sue is not unusual: I have had many people tell me diabetes is the best thing that ever happened to them. It caused them to develop a healthier lifestyle that increased energy levels, improved sleeping patterns and promoted weight loss.

The diagnosis of type 2 diabetes is an *invitation* to wellness and improved quality of life. It causes us to take a good look at ourselves and evaluate the things that are important to us.

Sugar Is *Not* the Problem!

Sugar, or glucose, works in the human body as gasoline works in an automobile. If your car runs out of gas, it stops. If we humans truly run out of sugar, we die. It's *how much* sugar we have in our blood at any given moment that makes the difference between health and diabetes complications.

Each human body must have a minimum amount of sugar in the blood at all times to stay alive. Humans are a lot more important and complex than automobiles are. We were created with a built-in reserve gas tank called the liver. When we eat food, our body changes that food into sugar.

The foods that turn into 100% sugar are carbohydrate foods. When we eat carbohydrate foods, it's like pulling up to the gas station and filling up the gas tank.

Every time we eat, the liver takes up about one-third of the meal and stores it in the form of glycogen. If our body begins to run low on fuel (sugar), the liver changes the stored glycogen into glucose and refuels us without our even eating. That causes the blood-sugar levels to go up, even though nothing has passed our lips.

It is natural to think, "If I don't eat, my blood sugar will go down."

Not so!

If we don't eat, our reserve gas tank, the liver, will kick out extra sugar to keep us going. This is a huge problem for people who have diabetes.

It is as important to eat enough as it is not to eat too much!

Type 2 diabetes is a fuel-injection problem. People who don't have diabetes have a built-in *balancer* that keeps the blood sugar between 65 mg/dl and 140 mg/dl most of the time, even if they eat a whole German chocolate cake. If their blood sugar goes up, the pancreas makes more insulin, which keeps the blood sugar from going too high. When the blood sugar reaches the normal range, the pancreas quits making extra insulin. If their blood sugar starts to drop too low, the liver changes glycogen into sugar and pumps it into the blood to keep the sugar level from going too low. When the blood sugar reaches the normal range again, the liver quits making extra sugar. This is how people who don't have blood-sugar issues maintain healthy sugar balance all the time.

If a person has type 2 diabetes, however, their *balancer* is broken. When their blood sugar begins to drop because they have not eaten the correct amount of fuel food at the right time, the liver kicks out extra sugar; unfortunately, the broken balancer cannot always shut the liver off once the blood sugar returns to normal levels. This is bad news for someone who has diabetes, because the liver can keep causing the sugar to go up, up, up. At this point, we wish the pancreas could produce enough insulin to keep the rising sugar in check—it can't. The *balancer* is broken.

So what *can* people with type 2 diabetes do? *They* become their *own* balancer! They have to balance the blood sugar from the outside-in by the choices they make. It is about maintaining a constant fuel level throughout their waking hours. They can do this in the following ways:

1) Eating the correct amount of carbohydrate at the correct time each day
2) Exercising at the correct time in relation to eating meals or snacks
3) Managing stress levels

For those of us old enough to have driven a car that had a carburetor, we know what happened when the carburetor flooded! It stopped, and the car was not going anywhere until the excess gas drained completely out of the carburetor. Our body is like that carburetor. If we flood our body by eating more fuel food than our body needs, it will cough and sputter and keep going as long as it can, but eventually our body will need a tow truck. We can easily avoid the tow truck by becoming our body's own *balancer.* It is easier than you might think!

Type 2 diabetes is a lifestyle disease

People who have type 2 diabetes have insulin resistance. Insulin is the hormone that makes it possible to maintain healthy blood-sugar levels. When we eat, our blood sugar naturally goes up. When blood sugar goes up, the pancreas produces insulin. Insulin is the key that unlocks the pathways through the cell wall so sugar may enter the cell. This happens to trillions of cells at the same time, which makes it possible for the body to be fed, or fueled.

Insulin fits into cell receptors in order to unlock the fuel pathways. If insulin cannot enter the receptors, sugar is locked out of the cell. If the blood sugar cannot enter the cells because the insulin cannot unlock the pathways, the blood sugar just keeps going higher and higher. This is called *insulin resistance.*

There are four common choices we humans make for ourselves that increase insulin resistance:

1. Our food choices
    If I were to find myself out on the road, unprepared for a snack or meal, and I chose to eat a really "fast" meal—a sandwich with two meat patties, fries, and a milk shake—I

would greatly increase my body's insulin resistance.

Let's take a look at the fats in that meal: two meat patties, two cheese slices, a quarter of a cup of sauce, fries cooked in grease, and high-fat ice cream and milk. That is a ton of fat!

Now, let's look at the carbohydrate content of that meal: three slices of bread (large bun), potatoes, milk and ice cream. That is a ton of carbohydrate!

That meal, my friends, would be an assault on my body. My liver—the largest digestive organ in the body—would have to deal with that assault. My liver would do the best it could, but when it has to sort out a meal like that, it produces a by-product called *triglycerides*.

Triglycerides are free-floating fat globules in the blood that can prevent the insulin (a key) from unlocking the cell pathways, by keeping the insulin out of the receptor sites (the locks). If the insulin cannot unlock the pathways, the cells cannot be fed and the sugar stays outside of the cells in the circulating blood. Blood-sugar levels get higher and higher. Think of this like stuffing chewed bubblegum into a lock—it might be a perfectly good lock and a perfectly good key, but if the lock is full of bubblegum, it won't work very efficiently. If I ate that meal, the large amount of carbohydrates would cause my blood sugar to go way up, and the high fat content would make it difficult for my insulin to do its job of moving sugar into my cells. This would cause my blood sugar to remain high for a very long time.

> *The foods we choose to eat have a direct impact on the degree of insulin resistance we have. This directly affects our blood-sugar levels.*

2. The exercise we do or do not do

There is a *glut-4 transporter* in every muscle cell that moves the fuel (sugar) from the loading dock on the cell wall into the cell mitochondria, which are the powerhouses of the cell. This transporter takes sugar from the blood and makes it available to the muscles for energy. Fuel is burned in the mitochondria and changed into energy which makes it possible for us to live, move, and do.

My neighbor to the north runs five miles every morning. He is burning a lot of sugar! I have another friend, who has a common self-diagnosed allergy--*he is allergic to exercise*. About the most exercise he gets is clicking the remote on football nights. Is he burning sugar? Absolutely! He would not be able to move his thumb if he didn't have sugar to fuel his thumb muscles. Is he burning very much sugar? Absolutely *not*!

There was a study done several years ago checking into the work of glut-4 transporters. This study showed that people like my neighbor to the north who exercise regularly have a whole fleet of glut-4 transporters in every muscle cell and that people like my friend who is "allergic" to exercise are lucky to have *one* transporter in each muscle cell. So who do you think has the easier time maintaining healthy blood-sugar levels? Definitely the exerciser!

The exercise we choose to do or not do has a direct impact on the degree of insulin resistance we have. This directly affects our blood-sugar levels.

3. The amount of weight we carry on our body.
   If we carry unnecessary weight, muscle cells are packed tight with fat cells. This makes it difficult for insulin to squeeze into the receptors and unlock the cell pathways. If cell pathways cannot be unlocked, the cell cannot be fed. Sugar then remains in the blood, getting higher and higher. Insulin resistance greatly increases.

Allowing our body to carry unnecessary weight has a direct impact on the degree of insulin resistance we have. This directly affects our blood-sugar levels.

4. Stress!
   When I was a Neanderthal lady and saw a saber-toothed tiger salivating in the bushes, thinking he was about to have a juicy lady for lunch, my heart skipped a beat—I did *not* want to be his lunch. My body began to produce cortisol, adrenalin, and glucagon.

My heart beat faster; I breathed faster and more shallow. My muscles tensed, and my heart rate and blood pressure went up. My liver, the reserve fuel tank, began to pump out lots of extra sugar. All this happened to prepare me to run like the dickens, and run I did. My muscles burned up all the extra sugar my liver could pump out.

Finally, I got back to the cave. "Whew, that was way too close for comfort!"

Deep breath...Relax! All those helpful emergency hormones went back to normal. My blood pressure was normal. My breathing and heart rate were normal. My muscles relaxed, and my liver stopped making extra sugar.

Thankfully, *all* was back to normal!

All of us have saber-toothed tigers in our lives today—they just don't salivate. Maybe it's traffic we have to contend with; maybe it's a challenging child or spouse, a contentious boss, or a mortgage we don't know how we're going to pay. Whatever it is, our bodies react the very same way they did when we truly had to escape saber-toothed tigers: our blood sugar goes up, our blood pressure goes up, our heart and breathing rates go up, and our muscles are tensed.

The problem is that not very many people ever get back to the cave. We don't relax! Many of us live with constant stress, which we call *chronic stress syndrome*. We have high blood pressure, we have high blood sugar, and we have heart and muscle problems. We are *not* healthy.

Stress elevates emergency hormones, which have a direct impact on the degree of insulin resistance we have. This directly affects our blood-sugar levels. If we want to live well with diabetes, we must choose to eat well, exercise well, and manage stress well. After that, it's a piece of cake...just sayin'!

Remember these three basic principles:

1. **Healthy Eating.** Eat the right amount of fuel food at the right time. Carbohydrate must be

counted by the meal and the snack. Carbohydrate can *never* be counted by the day.

2. **Regular Exercise.** Always exercise with a full fuel tank. *Never* exercise on empty.

Exercise after a meal or snack. If you exercise on empty, your liver will have no choice but to produce extra sugar.

3. **Good Stress Management.** Schedule time every day to relax. Plan time to reduce stress levels.

Managing stress does not happen by accident. Make sure your diabetes self-management plan includes a stress-management plan.

Small, simple choices in these three areas can make a world of difference in how one feels, how one thinks, how one acts and reacts, and how one experiences life.

Know Your Opponent

Diabetes is ugly, ruthless, and mean. It is no respecter of persons. It doesn't care whether you are rich or poor; whether you are young or old; whether you are red, yellow, black, or white; or whether you are female or male. Even children as young as four years old are now being diagnosed with type 2 diabetes.

If you have diabetes and do not manage it, diabetes will manage you. The outcome will not be pretty. Diabetes left to itself is the number-one cause of adult blindness, the number-one cause of kidney failure requiring dialysis, and the number-one cause of non-traumatic amputation.

People who have *unmanaged* diabetes are two to four times more likely to have a heart attack or a stroke when compared to people who do not have diabetes.

Diabetes is the silent disabler. Once a person develops symptoms of diabetes complications, it is usually too late to correct the problem. The patient and his or her medical team may be able to stop the complication so it doesn't continue to get worse, but it most often cannot be reversed. Diabetes self-management is about prevention, prevention, and *more* prevention!

The medical profession has known about diabetes since the Egyptians built the pyramids, but it wasn't until 1993 that we finally figured out that diabetes complications can be prevented with simple self-management choices. Until then, we believed anyone unfortunate enough to be diagnosed with diabetes eventually would develop serious eye disease, suffer from kidney disease, endure an amputation, and possibly even suffer a heart attack or stroke.

So what changed? The 1993 report from the Diabetes Control and Complication Trial indicated that diabetes complications could be prevented by keeping blood-sugar levels closer to normal. In 1998, the United Kingdom Prospective Diabetes Study supported that conclusion.

According to the National Institute of Diabetes and Digestive and Kidney Diseases and the American Diabetes Association's 2012 statistics, people ages twenty and older who are affected by diabetes in the United States include the following:

* More than 10% of women
* More than 11% of men
* Nearly 16% of American Indians and Alaskan Native Americans
* Nearly 15% of African Americans
* Nearly 13% of Hispanic and Latino Americans
* Nearly 9% of Asian Americans
* Nearly 8% of non-Hispanic white Americans

When we look at a group of people and know that probably one of every ten persons in that group has diabetes, it boggles the mind. Then, to realize one of each three of the remaining nine people is estimated to have *prediabetes*, it feels overwhelming!

(Prediabetes is discussed in the chapter "In the Nick of Time.")

In 2013, diabetes was the seventh leading cause of death by disease in the United States. Heart attack was the first leading cause of death, and stroke was the fourth. We know unmanaged diabetes greatly increases the risk for heart attack and stroke. It is clear that diabetes can be a very dangerous opponent in the face of impending death. The good news is that, in today's world, we have all the tools and information we need to live well with diabetes. The choice is up to each one of us!

The Path of Destruction

Red blood cells are the part of the blood that carry oxygen to all other living cells in the body. Without oxygen, life cannot be sustained, so red blood cells have an extremely important job to do.

When red blood cells travel along in the bloodstream with all the other things blood carries, a little bit of sugar attaches to the outside of the red blood cells. This is a normal process called *glycosylation*. This is not a problem if the blood sugar is constantly in normal ranges; however, if the blood sugar is higher than it should be, more and more sugar begins to attach to the outside of the red cells, and they become sugar-coated—crispy, crunchy, crusty critters. Dr. Oz has referred to them as "shards of glass."

Once sugar has attached to the red cell, we don't know how to get it off of the red cell. The sugar will remain attached for the cell's entire lifetime. A red cell lives for about 90 days, or three months. The body is constantly producing new red cells every day to take the place of the red cells that are dying off. That's why many physicians measure the percentage of sugar attached to red cells once every three months. A blood test called an A1C measures the percentage of sugar coating on red cells. If I get my A1C checked today, my youngest, healthiest red cell will be dead in three months— so if I measure A1C every three months, I am measuring a whole new crop of red cells. The American Diabetes Association recommends that people with diabetes who are meeting treatment goals and have stable blood glucose levels have the A1C test twice a year. Health care providers may repeat the A1C test as often as four times a year until blood glucose reaches recommended levels.

The reason crispy critters are such a problem has to do with circulation. Normal, healthy red cells are very pliable and soft. They can squeeze, bend, and stretch to get through the smallest blood vessel in order to take oxygen to whatever is depending on it for a supply. If I have crispy critters in my blood, that is a major problem. Crispy critters may not be able to squeeze through a microscopic blood vessel (also known as a capillary) in fact, crispy critters may clog those smallest blood vessels. If that happens, the organs of the body that depend on microscopic capillaries for their life-giving supplies are out of luck. If red cells cannot get through with oxygen, neither can serum get through with nutrition. When that happens to enough body cells at one time, it will cause tissue damage, and when there's enough tissue damage, organ damage occurs. Remember, the organs that are primarily affected by this problem are the eyes (number-one cause of adult blindness), the kidneys (number-one cause of kidney failure requiring dialysis), and the nerves (number-one cause of non-traumatic amputation).

Unmanaged diabetes is a disaster!

When crispy critters flow through the larger blood vessels—the ones you can see with your naked eye—they scrape the inside lining of those blood vessels. Where there is a scrape, an inflammation occurs; where there is an inflammation, a scab forms. That scab becomes a cholesterol magnet, and atherosclerotic plaque begins to form. If the plaque builds up to the point where it completely occludes, or blocks, the blood vessel, and it's in your brain, it's called a stroke; if it is in your heart, it's called a heart attack. If the occlusion is in your legs or feet, it can cause gangrene, and there is only one way to treat gangrene—chop it off!

I can't emphasize enough that diabetes is mean and ugly and ruthless. It doesn't care if you're rich or poor; red, yellow, black, or white; a doctor or a cab driver—if you have diabetes and do not manage it, diabetes will manage you, and it won't be a pretty sight.

Eye. The eye works like a camera. If I am looking at a tree, light will carry the image of the tree through the lens of my eye and imprint the image on my retina. The retina is a thin layer of nerve cells that lines the inside of the eye and communicates with the brain by way of the optic nerve.

It's my brain that identifies the image of the tree and lets me know what I'm seeing. The retina gets all of its oxygen and nutrition through teeny, tiny microscopic blood vessels. If those blood vessels become clogged because I have crispy critters flowing along in my bloodstream, my eye is in big trouble. The retina tries to correct this problem by growing its own bypasses, tiny extra blood vessels—a process called *proliferative retinopathy*. The problem is that the new bypass blood vessels are weak, puny, and fragile and tend to rupture very easily, especially if there are crispy critters trying to flow through them. If they rupture and bleed into the chamber of the eye, light cannot pass through blood, and that will cast a shadow on the retina. The brain will say, "Hmmm, dark spot, field of vision."

And that, my friends, is diabetes eye disease!

Kidney. Kidneys filter between 120 and 150 quarts of blood each day. The kidneys' job is to allow waste to go out through the urine and to keep the "good stuff" in the body, by redirecting it back into the body's blood supply. The kidneys' filters are called *nephrons*. There are about one million microscopic nephrons in each kidney.

Imagine each nephron being made out of cheesecloth. The blood flows into the nephrons, allowing the waste to flow out with the urine and the good stuff to be circulated back into the bloodstream. Cheesecloth is a very fragile fabric. If I have normal blood-sugar levels, the blood flowing into those fragile nephrons is very nephron-friendly. However, if I have crispy critters flowing into my nephrons, those crispy critters will begin to tear the fabric—enlarging the holes in the filters through which the waste flows. That will allow some of the good stuff to escape through the urine. The first thing that gets through is microalbumin—a protein that should remain in the body's blood supply. There is a test for urine microalbumin that is one of the routine lab tests for someone who has diabetes. If I have crispy critters *and* high blood pressure, the cheesecloth (my nephrons) will tear twice as fast. Diabetes is the number-one cause of kidney failure requiring dialysis; high blood pressure is the number-two cause of kidney failure. The combination of diabetes and high blood pressure is kidney suicide.

Nerves. The nervous system includes the brain, or main computer, and the nerves, a network of pathways that relays information through-out the body. Our brain is in charge of ordering and maintaining the functions of the body. The nerves make it possible for the brain to maintain two-way communication with the various parts of the body. This communication system makes it possible for the brain to maintain healthy control of all bodily functions.

Have you ever experienced corroded battery cables on your car? When the battery cables are corroded, the battery cannot send a spark to the combustion engine to get the motor started. The communication between the battery and the engine is blocked. If my blood sugar is higher than it should be, my nerves can become corroded with sugar, which can cause an interruption in the communication between the body parts and the brain.

It is the brain that communicates to the muscles of the foot what shape the foot needs to maintain. If the nerves are corroded, the muscles may not know in what shape to keep the foot, which could result in a condition called *Charcot foot*. Charcot foot is a serious complication of unmanaged diabetes.

If the nerve pathways become corroded, it may cause strange sensations in various parts of the body, such as tingling, burning, stinging, the feeling of insects crawling, or even a complete loss of feeling in the feet, the hands, or both. Nerve pathways communicate to the digestive system how the stomach and intestines should process food. Another serious complication of unmanaged diabetes is *gastroparesis*, or paralysis of the stomach.

Years ago, a patient shared that he had slipped off a curb and sprained his ankle on the way home from work one evening. He went to the emergency room. The doctor came into his cubicle and said, "The good news is that your ankle is not broken. But look at this!"

The doctor then put the X-ray on the reader, and it showed that he had a thumbtack in his heel that had been there so long the skin had grown over the top. He had to have the thumbtack surgically removed. He had had type 2 diabetes for about fifteen years; he took his medication as prescribed and thought that was all he needed to do—that the medication would keep him healthy.

He didn't understand that keeping his blood sugar in healthy levels required his participation, and as a result, his blood sugar was always higher than normal. Over time, he had lost all feeling in his feet and could not feel the tack when he stepped on it.

I wanted to know why he didn't get an infection. He said the doctor had the same question and decided that he had had such a thick callus on his heel that the tack never reached the foot tissue.

With normal nerve function in his foot, he would have felt the tack when he stepped on it. He was very fortunate: had he developed an infection, he may have ended up with an amputated foot or leg.

Sugar is carried in the blood. Blood *must* touch every living cell in the body in order for it to stay alive and well. This means *nothing* in the human body can escape the harmful effects of high blood sugar. It is each individual's responsibility to make healthy choices to keep him- or herself alive and well. There is no medication in the world that will manage type 2 diabetes. Many television ads for type 2 diabetes medication include the phrase "along with diet and exercise." Diabetes is a lifestyle disease. Medication, if needed, *helps* us live well with diabetes—it does not cure or manage type 2 diabetes.

What's the Game Plan?

Maintaining healthy blood-sugar levels in the face of diabetes is all about fuel injection. Sugar to the human body is like gasoline to an automobile. If the car gets sporadic bursts of barely enough gas or too much gas, it coughs and sputters and chugs along until it can go no farther. Our bodies act pretty much the same unless we can fuel them in nice, even increments throughout our waking hours. We begin fueling our bodies correctly by recognizing the "fuel foods," or carbohydrates. Carbohydrates are foods that turn into 100 percent sugar even though they may not contain any sugar. Carbohydrates are *not* bad foods—they're essential foods. When we eat carbohydrates, it's like pulling up to the gas station and filling up the gas tank. Fuel foods include milk, yogurt, fruit, fruit juice, bread, cereal, rice, pasta, potatoes, peas, corn, sweet potatoes, acorn squash, butternut squash, spaghetti squash, all dried beans, and anything made of any kind of flour.

A good rule of thumb for measuring *one carbohydrate choice* is to measure half of a cup for most of the foods listed above and one-third of a cup for rice and pasta. All cooked foods are measured after they have been cooked. Any fresh fruit the size of a baseball is one choice; if it is larger than a baseball, it is two choices. Oranges need to be measured after they are peeled. I find that clementine oranges count as one choice for my body requirements. Melons are cut into bite-size pieces, and one level measuring cup constitutes one choice. Most berries are one cup. Fruit is really quick sugar—never eat two fruit choices at one time. That would be too much quick sugar all at once.

When we eat carbohydrate choices, it is important to remember we can eat more later for the next snack or meal—we do not have to eat it all right now!

These foods need to be eaten at the right time and in the right amount. If we eat too few carbohydrate choices, our liver has to make extra sugar—that throws our bodies out of balance. If we eat too many carbohydrate choices, we flood the carburetor, and *that* throws our bodies out of balance. It is up to each individual to balance his body from the outside-in by making correct carbohydrate choices—the right amounts at the right times.

The first fuel stop of the day is breakfast—this is true for everyone, whether you work during the day or during the night. Breakfast counts as the first meal you eat after your longest period of sleep and is extremely important. It needs to be eaten within thirty minutes of getting out of bed.

At this point, the body has gone its longest period of time without food. When you get out of bed, your muscles need to move, but your body is out of fuel. If you fail to feed your body, your muscles will send out "we need fuel" messages, and your liver will begin to change glycogen into glucose, causing your blood sugar to go up even though you didn't eat anything. This process happens so your muscles can have the fuel they need to continue moving.

The liver can be a wonderful emergency fuel reserve for people who do not have blood-sugar issues. For people who do have blood-sugar issues, however, the liver can cause a disaster. People who have blood-sugar issues want to keep their liver content, happy, and never needing to help.

Eating breakfast within thirty minutes of getting out of bed keeps the liver from dumping more sugar into the bloodstream. Beginning with breakfast, meals and snacks should be eaten at regular intervals throughout your waking hours. Meals and snacks should be eaten no closer than 2 hours apart, and no further than 4 hours apart. For example, if I eat breakfast at 7:00 a.m., I will eat a snack at 10:00 a.m., lunch at 1:00 p.m., a snack at 4:00 p.m., dinner at 7:00 p.m., and if needed, a snack before bed at 10:00 p.m. This schedule will provide my body with nice, even fuel injection. It will keep my liver content and *not* helping!

It is as important to eat enough carbo-hydrate as it is not to eat too much!

If we fail to eat enough carbohydrate during our waking hours, the liver will have no choice but to pour sugar into the bloodstream in the middle of the night to keep our body adequately fueled. One way to know whether this is happening is to check your blood sugar 2 hours after dinner or at bedtime and again first thing the next morning. If your evening blood sugars are lower than your morning numbers, your body has run out of fuel during the night and your liver has had to start producing sugar to keep your body functioning. If you eat the correct amount of carbohydrate the day before, your body will have an adequate supply of fuel to keep your body functioning all night. Your blood-sugar level will gradually go down as you sleep, and your morning blood-sugar levels will be lower than they were when you went to bed—hence the need to eat breakfast within thirty minutes of getting up!

What is a carbohydrate choice?

We measure gasoline by the gallon. We measure carbohydrate by the "choice." One gallon is equal to four quarts of gas; one carbohydrate choice contains exactly 15 grams of carbohydrate. There aren't very many foods that come in exactly 15 grams of carbohydrate. If we round it off, anything that contains 15–22 grams of carbohydrate can be counted as one choice (closer to 15 than to 30) and anything that contains 23–37 grams of carbohydrate can be counted as two choices (closer to 30 than to 15). Thirty grams of carbohydrate would be exactly two choices. If we eat something that contains more than 37 grams of carbohydrate, we have to divide the total number of carbohydrate by 15 to find out how many choices it contains. For example, a raisin bagel that contains 58 grams of carbohydrate would be four choices. (Rounding 58 up to 60 and dividing by 15 equals four choices.)

When reading Nutrition Facts labels, there are only two things to look at with regard to blood sugar:

1. What is the recommended *serving size*, which can be found right under the words *Nutrition Facts*?
2. How much *total carbohydrate* will you eat if you eat one recommended serving?

*You do not need to look at **Sugars** ever. Sugar is a carbohydrate and will be included in the "total carbohydrate" number on the Nutrition Facts label.*

For example, a recommended serving size for Honey Nut Cheerios is three-quarters of a cup; this would equal 22 grams of carbohydrate which would be counted as one choice. Three-quarters of a cup of Cheerios is not a bowl of cereal! If I ate one cup of Cheerios, I would get nearly 29 grams of carbohydrate which would be two carbohydrate choices—one cup is still *not* a bowl of cereal. One carbohydrate choice more than your body can process has the potential to raise your blood sugar 50 points. It is important to carefully measure your carbohydrate choices!

Another source of carbohydrate choices comes in the form of beverages. For example, a 20 FL OZ bottle of Sprite contains 26 grams of carbohydrate per serving; there are 2.5 servings per bottle—78 grams of carbohydrate or five choices per bottle. A bottle of V•Fusion contains 42 grams of carbohydrate—three choices. A F'real 10 FL OZ vanilla milkshake contains 73 grams of carbohydrate—five choices. Please be aware that it is extremely important to check the total carbohydrate content of anything you plan to swallow—*all* foods and drinks that contain carbohydrate *must* be included in the carbohydrate meal plan.

Some foods we eat will not cause our blood sugar to go up. We refer to these foods as "freebies." Nonstarchy and leafy green vegetables do not have enough carbohydrate to even count. Some examples of these foods are carrots, tomatoes, broccoli, cauliflower, asparagus, green beans, spinach, zucchini, yellow summer squash, cucumbers, celery, mushrooms, onions, peppers, cabbage, kale, and all salad greens. You can eat as much of these foods as you want, whenever you want, without causing your blood sugar to go up.

Remember you can eat freebies anytime.

Men of moderate physical activity need three to four choices for each of three meals per day and one to two choices for each of three snacks per day. This is a beginning point. If a man is very sedentary, he may not need that much; he could eat three choices for a meal and one choice for a snack—but no fewer carbohydrates than that. If a man is very active, he may need to increase his carbohydrate intake a little. Monitoring blood sugar with a glucose meter will help you decide whether you need more or fewer carbohydrates to keep your blood sugar in balance.

Women of moderate physical activity need three choices for each of three meals per day and one choice for each of three snacks per day. This is a beginning point. A woman may eat as few as two choices for each meal and one choice for each snack, but no fewer. Again, it is as important to eat enough carbohydrate as it is not to eat too much.

The other group of foods that do not elevate blood sugar is the proteins: meat, fish, poultry, eggs, cheese, nuts, and peanut butter. A whole serving of meat, fish, or poultry after being baked, grilled, or broiled is the size of a single deck of cards. One egg, one ounce of cheese, one-fourth cup of nuts, and two tablespoons of peanut butter equal one serving. Even though proteins do not raise blood sugar, they contain fats, which can cause two things:

1) If we eat too much fat, we get fat.
2) If we eat too much fat, it makes it hard for our body to use its own (or injected) insulin.

Eating too much fat increases insulin resistance. Meals usually consist of a variety of carbohydrate and protein. Proteins come with fat. The carbohydrates raise our blood sugar, and if we have eaten too much protein, the fat in the protein will keep the blood sugar from coming down. That leaves too much sugar in the blood for a longer period of time.

The longer we have higher levels of blood sugar, the higher our A1C will be and the higher our risk for developing complications will be.

You can use the following *Personal Meal Plan* form to design a basic meal plan for yourself. Once you have a basic plan, you can exchange carbohydrate foods of equal value within the plan for variety. It is most important to eat the correct amount of fuel food (carbohydrate) at the correct times throughout your waking hours. *Be sure to eat some protein at each meal and snack.* Remember, meals or snacks cannot be closer than two hours apart, and they cannot be further apart than four hours.

Personal Meal Plan

Time_____ get out of bed: (eat breakfast within 30 minutes of getting up)

Time_____ breakfast: (Women 2 – 3 choices, Men 3 – 4 choices)

Time_____ snack: (Women 1 choice, Men 1 – 2 choices)

Time_____ lunch: (Women 2 – 3 choices, Men 3 – 4 choices)

Time_____ snack: (Women 1 choice, Men 1 – 2 choices)

Time_____ dinner: (Women 2 – 3 choices, Men 3 – 4 choices)

Time_____ bedtime snack: (Women 1 choice, Men 1 – 2 choices)

Time_____ go to bed

*One carbohydrate choice rounded off
equals 10–22 grams (precisely 15 grams).
Be sure to pair carbohy-
drates with protein.
Exchange carbohydrate foods of equal
value within the plan for variety!*

Personal Meal Plan (Sample: Woman)

Time___6:30___get out of bed: (eat breakfast within 30 minutes of getting up)

Time__7:00__breakfast: (*Women 2 – 3 choices*, Men 3 – 4 choices)

> Egg—protein: free
> Small orange: 1 choice
> Whole-wheat English muffin: 2 choices
> Coffee with one tablespoon flavored creamer: free

Time 10:00 snack: (*Women 1 choice*, Men 1 – 2 choices)

> Apple: 1 choice
> Peanut butter—protein: free

Time 1:00 lunch: (*Women 2 – 3 choices*, Men 3 – 4 choices)

> Ham sandwich, tomato, lettuce, cheese, mustard: 2 choices
> and protein (ham): free
> Chips: 1 choice
> Unsweetened tea: free

Time <u>4:00 </u>**snack:** *(Women 1 choice, Men 1 – 2* **choices)**

> Cheese—protein: free
> Crackers: 1 choice
> Unsweetened tea: free

Time <u>7:00 </u>**dinner:** *(Women 2 – 3 choices,* **Men 3 – 4 choices)**

> Chicken—protein: free
> Three-inch baked potato: 2 choices
> Butter and sour cream—fat: free
> Green salad: free
> Broccoli: free
> One cup milk: 1 choice

thirty minutes walking after dinner

Time <u>10:00 </u>**bedtime snack:** *(Women 1 choice,* **Men 1 – 2 choices)**

> Peanut butter—protein: free
> 2 graham cracker squares: 2/3 choice
> 1/2 cup milk: 1/3 choice

Time <u>10:30 </u>**go to bed**

One carbohydrate choice rounded off equals 10–22 grams (precisely 15 grams). Be sure to pair carbohydrates with protein. Exchange carbohydrate foods of equal value within the plan for variety!

Hunger is not part of the program!

If you have eaten all of your carbohydrate allowance for a particular meal or snack and are still hungry, you can eat all the freebies you want from the leafy-green and nonstarchy-vegetable group—even a little more protein, if you want. Only the carbohydrate foods directly affect the blood-sugar levels and need to be eaten in measured amounts at the right times.

When you eat with even fuel injection, two things happen:

1. Your blood sugar levels out. Your body no longer has to depend on its liver glycogen stores to fuel itself.
2. Your body will allow you to lose weight.

If we don't eat enough fuel food, our brain thinks either that our throats have been cut or that there is a famine in the land. This causes our body's metabolism to slow to a creep—everything gets turned into storage.

Storage is a three-letter word: F-A-T. Until we get our eating back into balance, our body will not turn loose of our fat stores. Our brain will believe we might have to live off those fat stores someday and will not allow us to lose even an ounce of weight.

Once we begin to eat healthily again, our metabolism can pick up and the body will begin to turn loose of its fat stores. I know it is counterintuitive to think "I have to eat to keep my blood sugar from going up" and "I have to eat to lose weight."

Both statements are true!

Warning:

Blood-sugar levels usually balance out within three to six weeks of adopting a healthy lifestyle: [1] healthy nutrition, [2] regular exercise, and [3] good stress management. Sometimes when we achieve blood-sugar goals quickly and easily, our mind convinces us we *didn't really have diabetes that badly.* We begin to fall back into our old habits, and before long, we are looking at a much higher A1C, and our health-care provider is recommending medication or increases in medication.

*The mind is a powerful
thing. Be on guard!*

How Do I Know I'm Winning?

* **BFF**—Your blood glucose meter is your *Best Friend Forever.* This inexpensive and simple at-home test can let you know from day to day whether what you are doing is working. Your doctor will help you set goals to achieve your best personal-health results. Sometimes age, other health diagnoses, and varying circumstances will make it necessary to adjust the goal numbers. Generally speaking, the American Diabetes Association and the American Association of Clinical Endocrinologists have established goals for non-pregnant persons that work for most people who have type 2 diabetes.

1993 American Diabetes Association Goals

Before meals .... 80 – 130 mg/dl
Two hours after first
bite of a meal .... Less than 180 mg/dl
Hemoglobin A1C ...... Less than 7% (general goal)

Individuals should keep their A1C as low as possible without causing low blood-sugar levels.

2003 American Association of Clinical Endocrinologists

Before meals .... Less than 110 mg/dl
Two hours after first
bite of a meal .... Less than 140 mg/dl
Hemoglobin A1C ...... 6.5% or less
Individuals should keep their A1C as low as possible without causing low blood-sugar levels.

If you keep track of your blood-sugar levels with your BFF, you will be able to identify foods that cause your blood sugar to go up and foods that don't affect your blood sugar. This gives you the power to make adjustments in your food intake that will keep your blood sugar in goal range.

* **A1C**—Your A1C is your term report card. The hemoglobin A1C measures the amount of blood sugar that is attached to your red blood cells. The higher the average of your blood sugar, the higher your A1C result will be. The A1C provides a three-month average of blood-sugar levels. Again, we do not know how to get sugar off of a red cell; the sugar-coated red cells must die, taking the sugar with them, in order to lower the A1C. The A1C is reported by a percentage value, and it corresponds to a mg/dl value that is more like the number you get when you check your blood sugar with your personal meter. It is reported as estimated average glucose, or eAG. An A1C of 6.5% to 7% is like getting an A+ or an A on your term report card.

If your A1C is 6.5%, your eAG would be 140 mg/dl. If your A1C is 8.5%, your eAG would be

197 mg/dl. An A1C of more than 7% indicates that long-term complications are silently taking place in your body. Again, diabetes is the number-one cause of adult blindness, number-one cause of kidney failure requiring dialysis, and the number-one cause of non-traumatic amputation. People who have unmanaged diabetes are two to four times more likely to have a stroke or a heart attack than are people who do not have diabetes.

Estimated Average Glucose

A1C %	eAG mg/dl
6	126
6.5	140
7	154
7.5	169
8	183
8.5	197
9	212
9.5	226
10	240

In the Nick of Time

In 2002, a study called the Diabetes Prevention Program (DPP) let us know for the first time that it is possible to prevent or delay type 2 diabetes. The study was done with about three thousand people, all of whom had blood-sugar levels that were higher than normal but that weren't high enough to be diagnosed as diabetes. Slightly elevated blood sugar is also known as impaired glucose tolerance (IGT) or impaired fasting glucose (IFG). There were three groups involved with the study.

Group one was the control group. They received placebos (pills that did not contain any medication) and were given basic instruction in diet and exercise.

Group two were given metformin, which is a very good first-line diabetes medication. They were also given basic instruction in diet and exercise.

Group three was the lifestyle group. This group was taught (1) to eat correctly, (2) to exercise regularly—at least thirty minutes five times per week, and (3) to schedule time into their busy days to reduce stress—a planned stress-management program.

The DPP showed us that making healthier choices in nutrition, exercise, and stress management reduced the risk of developing type 2 diabetes by 58 percent—a sharp reduction. The metformin group also reduced the risk of developing type 2 diabetes, but their results were less dramatic.

As a nurse, I was sure the metformin group would come out ahead, but the lifestyle group exceeded expectations! Remember, there are no medications that take care of diabetes—type 2 diabetes is a lifestyle disease. You must choose to take care of yourself, and then add medication, *if needed*, to keep your blood sugar at healthy levels.

Dr. Michael Roizen, Chief Wellness Officer for the Cleveland Clinic and Chair of its Wellness Institute, says "our lifestyle choices and behaviors have far more impact on longevity and health than our genetic inheritance." Dr. Roizen shared that multicountry studies show that about 25 percent of how you age is in your genes, while 75 percent is your choices. We *can* and *must* choose health to allow us to have an enjoyable future.

The American Diabetes Association recommends that testing to detect prediabetes and type 2 diabetes be considered in adults without symptoms who are overweight or obese and have one or more additional risk factors for diabetes. In those without these risk factors, testing should begin at age forty-five.

The following are additional risk factors for prediabetes:

* Being physically inactive
* Having a parent, brother, or sister with diabetes

* Having a family background that is African American, Alaska Native, Native American, Asian American, Hispanic or Latino, or Pacific Islander
* Giving birth to a baby weighing more than nine pounds or being diagnosed with gestational diabetes—diabetes first found during pregnancy
* Having high blood pressure—140/90 mmHg or above—or being treated for high blood pressure
* Having HDL, or "good" cholesterol, below 35 mg/dL, or a triglyceride level above 150 mg/dL
* Having polycystic ovary syndrome, also called PCOS
* Having impaired fasting glucose (IFG) or impaired glucose tolerance (IGT) on previous testing
* Having other conditions associated with insulin resistance, such as severe obesity or a condition called *acanthosis nigricans*, characterized by a dark, velvety rash around the neck or armpits
* Having a history of cardiovascular disease

If we are identified as having prediabetes, we have the opportunity to make some healthy choices for ourselves and turn the trend around. If we are discovered *in the nick of time*, we don't *have* to develop type 2 diabetes!

Diagnostic Values

Normal Fasting Blood sugar (FBS)	Less than 100 mg/dl
Normal Hemoglobin A1C	4 % – 5.6%
Prediabetes FBS	100 mg/dl-125 mg/dl
Prediabetes Hemoglobin A1C	5.7% – 6.4%
Diabetes FBS	126 mg/dl or greater
Hemoglobin A1C	6.5% or greater

What If...

* **What if I get my type 2 diabetes under perfect control? Will I still have diabetes forever?**

  Yes, type 2 diabetes is forever. Many people manage their diabetes perfectly with nutrition, exercise, and stress management; however, if they stopped living their healthy lifestyle, diabetes is still there and would immediately rear its ugly head with a vengeance. (Remember, the mind is a powerful thing.) Diabetes is forever, and a healthy lifestyle must be forever also.

* **What if I want to have a glass of wine with dinner?**

Alcohol is recognized by the body as a toxic substance. The liver (there it is again) is the detox organ of the body. The liver has a multitude of jobs to do, but it is not a multi-tasking organ. When we take our first sip of wine, mixed drink, or beer, our liver goes into the detox closet, slams the door shut, and doesn't come out until all the alcohol is gone. The liver is unavailable to us until *all* of the alcohol is completely out of our body. This can be a problem, because the liver plays a big role in keeping our blood sugar in normal levels. It takes about one hour for a man's body to get rid of one drink. It takes about an hour and a half for a woman's body to get rid of one drink. If our blood sugar starts to go too low during that time, the liver is *not* available to add more sugar to bring the blood sugar back to normal range. Some people who experience dangerously low blood sugar do so while drinking alcoholic beverages.

One alcoholic drink can usually be enjoyed each day. It is important to have food in combination with an alcoholic beverage, as this will lessen the possibility of developing low blood sugar. More than one drink at a time will increase the time the liver will be unable to help with other necessary jobs: not good! Some diabetes medications have warnings on their containers to not mix them with alcohol. Please follow medication instructions.

* **What if I want to have dessert after dinner?**

When you plan to eat dessert after dinner, just eat "free" foods for the meal. For example, have meat, fish, or chicken; a big green salad and steamed broccoli; then order guilt-free dessert. Dessert is not a nutritious choice, but it is a feel-good food once in a while. It is not advisable to have dessert *all* the time, but it's not a problem to have it every so often, as long as we keep the total carbohydrate within the meal plan—we can't eat dessert in addition to our carbohydrate meal allowance.

If we are going to a birthday party or other celebration, plan for the dessert by eating free foods for the meal. This is really important information for making it through the holidays and other special occasions. It's worth the reminder, there's always tomorrow: you don't have to eat the whole thing right now! Keep in mind the consequences—*very good* consequences if we keep to our meal plan. *Very bad* consequences if we throw out the meal plan.

If we slip up, remember tomorrow is a new day, and we can get it back together very quickly. It works if you work it!

* **What if the weather is bad and I can't get outside to exercise?**

The type of exercise doesn't really matter. We just need to *move*. Setting the kitchen timer and walking in the house will work just fine—even putting on some music and dancing will be effective and fun. In another vein, cleaning house is exercise also. Just move!

* **What if my stomach is too heavy after I eat? Why can't I exercise before eating?**

  Exercising on an empty fuel tank will cause your liver to produce extra sugar, and your blood sugar will go up, even without eating. If it is uncomfortable to exercise after a meal, eat something light before exercise. For a woman, one carbohydrate choice (15–22 grams) will carry your body for thirty minutes of exercise; a man may need two choices (23–37 grams), depending on the level of exercise intensity. Remember to pair a small amount of protein with a carbohydrate each time you eat.

* **What if my blood sugar is higher in the morning than it was the evening before?**

  When your morning fasting blood sugar is higher than your after-meal blood sugar was the evening before, it is usually an indication that you did not eat enough fuel food (carbohydrate) the day before. Food is medicine—it is the most important medicine when trying to manage type 2 diabetes. Skimping on fuel causes your body to run low in the middle of the night, and then your liver has to produce extra sugar to keep your body going. Unfortunately, if you have diabetes, your balancer is broken, and the sugar may continue to climb higher than the normal range. Remember, it is as important to eat enough as it is not to eat too much.

* **What if I already have serious diabetes complications?**

Diabetes is the silent disabler. If a person has symptoms of eye disease, kidney disease, or nerve damage, it may be too late to correct the problem. The important thing is to *stop* the progress of the disease and save the health you currently enjoy. Even if you have been diagnosed with complications, you will be able to enjoy a far better life by following the three steps of diabetes management: (1) healthy nutrition, (2) regular exercise, and (3) good stress management. It is *never* too late to adopt a healthier lifestyle.

* **What if I have done everything possible and my blood sugar is still not in a healthy range?**

The good news is that we know how to live well with type 2 diabetes in the twenty-first century. Many people will be able to manage perfectly well with a healthy lifestyle. If that is not enough, our health-care providers can prescribe medication to assist us. If we can manage diabetes with just lifestyle, great! If we need pills to help us manage diabetes, super! If we need insulin or other injections to manage our diabetes, we must be grateful we have access to whatever it takes to keep our A1C within goal range—that's how we prevent complications and live well with diabetes.

* **What if I feel sick and cannot eat?**

If you are nauseated, it is still important to try to meet your fuel requirements. Sipping on regular ginger ale or other regular soda may be one way to fuel your body. Sipping a quarter of a cup over a half hour throughout your waking hours may work. It is important to keep track of your blood sugar. Blood sugar can rise if your body is sick—the liver produces extra sugar in an effort to give your body extra energy to combat the illness. Keeping your carbohydrate intake constant may help keep your liver from producing extra sugar. If you begin vomiting, it is important to contact your physician, especially if you are on diabetes medications. Dehydration can come quickly and can be a dangerous condition.

* **What if my knee hurts or another part of my body is complaining? Should I just press on with my exercise?**

Always listen to your body. Do *not* force a hurting body part to exercise without first consulting your health-care provider. You can move the body parts that don't hurt. Some people opt for pool exercises, which do not put a lot of stress on joints. There are many movements that can be done while sitting in a chair. Any movement is better than no movement.

* **What if my blood sugar is lower before I exercise and higher after exercise?**

This is an indication that you need to eat more carbohydrates before exercise. This is one good example why your meter is your BFF: you can determine the correct amount of fuel to eat before exercise without flooding your carburetor.

* **What if I've never eaten breakfast and don't want to start?**

Health is all about choice. I've explained the importance of eating within thirty minutes of getting out of bed and why not eating can cause problems for your blood-sugar levels. You have the information necessary to make a personal choice.

* **What if I experience signs and symptoms of low blood sugar when my blood sugar is at 80 mg/dl?**

The brain does not require insulin to gain access to sugar. This means your brain has to function at whatever level you are running your blood sugar. If your blood sugar is averaging 140 mg/dl or less, your brain is a happy camper. If your blood sugar is averaging 200–300 mg/dl, your brain is working in s-y-r-u-p. That might be like trying to run the "440" in thick mud up to your knees. Nevertheless, the brain adapts the best it can to functioning in syrup. When the blood sugar comes down, even to 80 mg/dl, the brain has to adjust to more normal blood-sugar levels—a kind of earthquake in the brain. This can cause symptoms of low blood sugar that one might expect from a level of 40–50 mg/dl.

Over time, your brain will adapt to normal blood sugars and once again be a happy camper. It is important to note that any time you feel symptoms of low blood sugar, you should eat one carbohydrate choice (15 grams CHO). *Don't overtreat*: give your brain a little time to adjust to healthier blood-sugar levels again. Headaches are common during this phase of bringing your blood sugar into a healthy range.

* **What if I already have proliferative retinopathy?**

  Your eye physician will be able to treat the condition somewhat. Treatment sometimes leaves scar tissue on the retina, which decreases overall vision, but the vision you have left can, hopefully, be protected. It is extremely important for you to adopt a healthy diabetes self-management program to prevent further damage.

* **What if I want to save some of my lunch carbohydrate choices so I can eat more at dinner?**

  You cannot save carbohydrate choices from one meal to add to another meal or snack. If you do that, you will be causing your liver to make sugar at one meal and flooding your carburetor at another. One carbohydrate choice more than your body can process has the potential to raise your blood sugar fifty points. Remember, successfully eating with diabetes is about fuel injection—nice, even fuel injection throughout the waking hours.

*   **What if my family member wants to take charge of me?**

Family members are usually motivated by love, concern, and fear. They want to keep you safe and with them for a long time. The fact is, family members cannot be the food police, the exercise police, or the stress-management police. Each individual is responsible for himself or herself. I can't blame someone else for my health complications: I am in charge of me!

Some people may find it very helpful to have an accountability partner. This accountability comes in the form of encouragement, *not* criticism. Remember, the person with diabetes is in charge—as difficult as it is for family members to watch a loved one harm himself, they can help only as much as he allows.

Diabetes really is a family disease, and hopefully each family will work together for the best possible outcome!

* **What if I overeat at a meal or a snack? Can I just skip carbohydrate choices at my next scheduled meal or snack?**

   If you overeat, it is important that you get right back on the plan at the next meal or snack. Do *not* skip carbohydrate choices at your next scheduled meal or snack. Your body processes what you eat in about two hours. If you had extra for lunch, the extra will have already been sent to storage before your next scheduled meal or snack. Storage is fat. If you skip carbohydrate, your metabolism may slow down even more, which makes it difficult to maintain a healthy weight. If you get off schedule, forgive yourself and hop back on schedule as soon as possible!

* **What if I eat out? How can I stay within my carbohydrate allowance then?**

   In today's world, this is very simple. Those who have smartphones can just Google the eatery, request nutrition facts information for the item you plan to eat, and feel assured that you can knowingly choose foods that will allow you to stay within your carbohydrate allowance. If you do not have a smartphone, you can request the nutrition information from the restaurant manager.

Beware the Jabberwock

JABBERWOCKY
Lewis Carroll

'Twas brillig, and the slithy toves
Did gyre and gimble in the wabe:
All mimsy were the borogoves,
And the mome raths outgrabe.
"Beware the Jabberwock, my son!
The jaws that bite, the claws that catch!
Beware the Jubjub bird, and shun
The frumious Bandersnatch!"
He took his vorpal sword in hand:
Long time the manxome foe he sought—

So rested he by the Tumtum tree,
And stood awhile in thought.
And, as in uffish thought he stood,
The Jabberwock, with eyes of flame,
Came whiffling through the tulgey wood,
And burbled as it came!
One, two! One, two! And
through and through
The vorpal blade went snicker-snack!
He left it dead, and with its head
He went galumphing back.
"And, has thou slain the Jabberwock?
Come to my arms, my beamish boy!
O frabjous day! Callooh! Callay!"
He chortled in his joy.

'Twas brillig, and the slithy toves
Did gyre and gimble in the wabe;
All mimsy were the borogoves,
And the mome raths outgrabe.

I love this nonsensical poem. It is so fun to read out loud! I include it in this final chapter because some of the information found on the web with regard to diabetes makes about as much sense as this ridiculous tongue-twisting poem.

Be cautious about where you get your wellness information.

Safe Sites for Good Diabetes Self-Management Information

American Association of Diabetes Educators
www.diabeteseducator.org

American Diabetes Association
www.diabetes.org

National Diabetes Education Program
ndep.nih.gov

National Diabetes Information
Clearing house
diabetes.niddk.nih.gov

Academy of Nutrition and Dietetics
www.eatright.org

Acknowledgments

Louise Hamwey, RN, MS
Nursing instructor, par excellence,
who encouraged her
students to develop and pursue writing skills.

Kelly Harvey, MS, RD/LD, CDE
An exceptional colleague who inspired the
development and implementation of an excellent
diabetes self-management program.

Katherine W. Hess, whose enthusiasm and
countless
hours of editing and encouragement made
this book possible.

All my patients, whose lives have been renewed
by implementing the principles put forth
in this book.

A sincere thank-you.

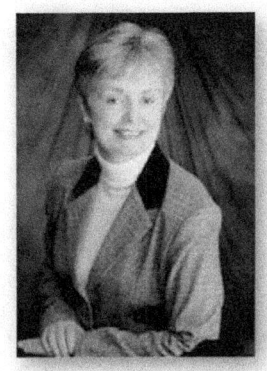

Carol J. Flick Wright, RN, CDE, was licensed to practice as a registered nurse in 1965. In 1994, she developed and implemented a self-management health-education program for a large internal-medicine and family-practice group. In 1996, she became a Certified Diabetes Educator. In 2000, she became a charter member of the board of directors for Maryland Foundation for Quality Healthcare, Inc. (MFQH). She wrote and implemented a diabetes self-management program for

MFQH that was awarded American Diabetes Association Recognition from November 2000 through November 2009. The MFQH Diabetes Self-Management Program received accreditation through the American Association of Diabetes Educators in December 2009. In 2011, Carol founded Diabetes Management, which provides individual diabetes and type 2 prevention counseling. She currently serves as the director and program coordinator for that organization.